THIS JOURNAL BELONGS TO

EMAIL _____

PHONE _____

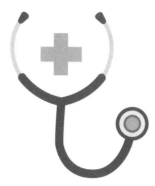

Published by Sourcebooks • P.O. Box 4410, Naperville, Illinois 60567-4410 • (630) 961-3900 • sourcebooks.com

Printed and bound in the United States of America.
VP 10 9 8 7 6 5 4 3 2 1

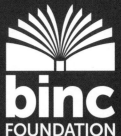

MY MEDICAL JO+RNAL

a **Practical Guide** with **Tips & Tricks**
for **Navigating** the **Medical Field** &
Logging Your Personal **Treatment Plan**

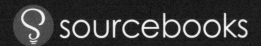

INTRODUCTION

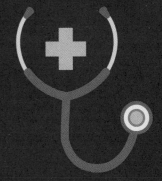

The information you collect can impact the quality of care you receive and help reduce the financial burden of your medical care. Sometimes medical providers may not record information accurately and the records you keep may have a big impact on your treatment and care.

- Use this journal to record all information on your medical care.
- Take the journal to all appointments and hospital stays.
- Ask questions and demand answers and explanations for anything you do not fully understand.
- Take another adult along to any visit to be the second set of ears.

- **Basic Information to record in this journal**
  - Contact information for each doctor or caregiver
  - Current list of medications
  - List of any allergies
  - Type and date of past surgeries, hospitalizations, and medical procedures
  - Record of each office or hospital visit

Copy and attach your
insurance card here.

Insurance Information

o PPO   o HMO   o Medicare   o Medicaid   Deductible $ _____

In-network % _____   Out of network % _____

Co-pay information _____

_____

_____

_____

_____

Provider Toll Free Phone _____

Referral needed for specialist?   o Yes   o No

Approval needed before procedure?   o Yes   o No

Copy and attach your Medicare/Medicaid

information on this page.

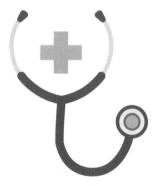

QUESTIONS
TO ASK

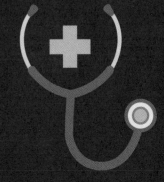

When choosing a doctor

QUESTIONS TO ASK

- Is my insurance accepted?
- What is "in-network" or "out-of-network" for my insurance?
  - Labs they use?
  - Affiliated hospital?
  - Physical Therapy/Occupational Therapy?
  - Referrals to other doctors?

- Is the practice owned by a hospital or licensed as a surgery center or independent practice? (Can lead to higher fees) Are "facility fees" or "visit fees" charged?
- Is there an APRN (Advanced Practice Registered Nurse), PA (Physician Assistant) or RN (Registered Nurse) available to answer questions?
- Are there lower charges for visits without doctor's interaction?
- What is their off-hours or on-call coverage?
- Are questions via phone or email accepted? Is there a charge? What is the normal response time?
- To what ER and/or hospital do they have admitting privileges?

**Always check with your insurance provider before treatments.
Make sure all referrals are "in-network".
If you are not able to afford medical care, see the
Negotiating Medical Bills section of this journal for
information on applying for charity care through the provider.**

When visiting a doctor's office

- Questions to ask about <u>tests, procedures & surgeries</u>
  - Why is this being ordered?
  - What results are expected?
  - Will having this test change my treatment plan?
  - What happens if we wait?
  - What is the cost?
  - Is a lower cost, less invasive alternative available?
  - Does the doctor. have a financial stake in the lab or clinic being used?

- Questions to ask about <u>medications & medical equipment</u>
  - What is the cost? Can equipment be rented? What will my insurance cover?
  - Is there a less expensive formulation/alternative with similar results?
  - What results should be expected? How long should it take to see results?
  - What side effects could arise? What to do if they occur?

- Ask the doctor or caregiver to spell, define, or explain anything you don't completely understand.

- What to record
  - Vitals at each visit (weight, blood pressure, etc.)
  - New treatments prescribed
  - New medications or therapy, or changes to existing
  - Answers to any of the above questions

Always check with your insurance provider with any questions about your coverage. Make sure all referrals are "in network".

In the hospital

- At check-in
  - Add "Consent is limited to in-network care only and excludes out-of-network care" or "Did not read" to any document you sign concerning your consent of financial responsibility.
  - Make sure you have a designated Power of Attorney.
  - What is your status upon admission? ("Admitted" or "For observation") What is the financial impact to you?

- During your stay
  - Ask for names and purpose of any doctor visiting your room. (If there is no purpose, you can refuse their visit and not be charged.)
  - What meds or treatments are they giving and why?

- At discharge
  - Be sure the discharge orders are appropriate for your home situation.
  - Will home care be needed? (Visiting Nurse, Home Care Aide, Therapist)

    How often and for how long?

    Can any of these services be out-patient instead?
    What is the cost? Covered by insurance?

  - Is any specialized equipment needed?

    What type?

    When will it be delivered?

    Have I received instructions for use?

    What will it cost? Covered by insurance?
    Do not accept any equipment you do not need or that can be inexpensively purchased or borrowed elsewhere. (i.e. wheelchairs, crutches, walkers) Local churches often have these items to loan.

- <u>Under the Affordable Care Act, nonprofit hospitals are required to provide free or discounted care to patients or risk losing their tax-exempt status.</u> Get contact information for the billing office and information on payment options for your financial situation.

Request forms and procedure for charity care, if needed.

**Always check with your insurance provider
with any questions about your coverage.**

Make sure all referrals are "in-network".

Before going to the pharmacy

CHECK ONLINE WEBSITES TO COMPARE PRICES AND FIND THE LEAST EXPENSIVE LOCAL PHARMACY.

- Goodrx.com
- Needymeds.org
- Singlecare.com

At the pharmacy

- Does the pharmacist know my all current meds, including over the counter medications, supplements, and vitamins?
- Is insurance prior-approval required?
- Will my insurance cover & what is my co-pay for new Rx?
- Is there any interaction or contraindication with other Rx I am taking?
- What results should be expected? How long should it take to see results?
- What side effects could arise? What to do if they occur?
- Is there an over the counter option?
- Is there a less expensive formulation or generic?
  - Will I need to appeal to my insurer for brand-name Rx?

Always check with your insurance provider with any questions about your coverage. Make sure all referrals are "in-network".

Pharmacy Notes

PHYSICIAN INFORMATION

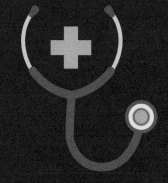

Doctor Name _____   Specialty _____

Assistant/PA Name _____   Off-hours Coverage _____

Phone Number _____

Email Address _____

Office Address _____

NOTES _____

_____

_____

_____

_____

_____

_____

Doctor Name _____   Specialty _____

Assistant/PA Name _____   Off-hours Coverage _____

Phone Number _____

Email Address _____

Office Address _____

NOTES _____

_____

_____

_____

_____

_____

_____

Doctor Name _____ Specialty _____

Assistant/PA Name _____ Off-hours Coverage _____

Phone Number _____

Email Address _____

Office Address _____

NOTES _____

_____

_____

_____

_____

_____

_____

Doctor Name _____ Specialty _____

Assistant/PA Name _____ Off-hours Coverage _____

Phone Number _____

Email Address _____

Office Address _____

NOTES _____

_____

_____

_____

_____

_____

_____

Doctor Name .... Specialty ....

Assistant/PA Name .... Off-hours Coverage ....

Phone Number ....

Email Address ....

Office Address ....

NOTES ....

....

....

....

....

....

....

Doctor Name .... Specialty ....

Assistant/PA Name .... Off-hours Coverage ....

Phone Number ....

Email Address ....

Office Address ....

NOTES ....

....

....

....

....

....

....

Doctor Name _____   Specialty _____

Assistant/PA Name _____   Off-hours Coverage _____

Phone Number _____

Email Address _____

Office Address _____

NOTES _____

_____

_____

_____

_____

_____

_____

_____

Doctor Name _____   Specialty _____

Assistant/PA Name _____   Off-hours Coverage _____

Phone Number _____

Email Address _____

Office Address _____

NOTES _____

_____

_____

_____

_____

_____

_____

_____

Doctor Name _____ Specialty _____

Assistant/PA Name _____ Off-hours Coverage _____

Phone Number _____

Email Address _____

Office Address _____

NOTES _____

_____

_____

_____

_____

_____

_____

_____

Doctor Name _____ Specialty _____

Assistant/PA Name _____ Off-hours Coverage _____

Phone Number _____

Email Address _____

Office Address _____

NOTES _____

_____

_____

_____

_____

_____

_____

Doctor Name _____   Specialty _____

Assistant/PA Name _____   Off-hours Coverage _____

Phone Number _____

Email Address _____

Office Address _____

NOTES _____

_____

_____

_____

_____

_____

_____

_____

_____

_____

Doctor Name _____   Specialty _____

Assistant/PA Name _____   Off-hours Coverage _____

Phone Number _____

Email Address _____

Office Address _____

NOTES _____

_____

_____

_____

_____

_____

_____

_____

_____

Doctor Name _____   Specialty _____

Assistant/PA Name _____   Off-hours Coverage _____

Phone Number _____

Email Address _____

Office Address _____

NOTES _____

_____

_____

_____

_____

_____

_____

_____

Doctor Name _____   Specialty _____

Assistant/PA Name _____   Off-hours Coverage _____

Phone Number _____

Email Address _____

Office Address _____

NOTES _____

_____

_____

_____

_____

_____

_____

Doctor Name _____ Specialty _____

Assistant/PA Name _____ Off-hours Coverage _____

Phone Number _____

Email Address _____

Office Address _____

NOTES _____

_____

_____

_____

_____

_____

_____

_____

_____

Doctor Name _____ Specialty _____

Assistant/PA Name _____ Off-hours Coverage _____

Phone Number _____

Email Address _____

Office Address _____

NOTES _____

_____

_____

_____

_____

_____

_____

_____

Doctor Name _____   Specialty _____

Assistant/PA Name _____   Off-hours Coverage _____

Phone Number _____

Email Address _____

Office Address _____

NOTES _____

_____

_____

_____

_____

_____

_____

Doctor Name _____   Specialty _____

Assistant/PA Name _____   Off-hours Coverage _____

Phone Number _____

Email Address _____

Office Address _____

NOTES _____

_____

_____

_____

_____

_____

Doctor Name _____   Specialty _____

Assistant/PA Name _____   Off-hours Coverage _____

Phone Number _____

Email Address _____

Office Address _____

NOTES _____

_____

_____

_____

_____

_____

_____

_____

Doctor Name _____   Specialty _____

Assistant/PA Name _____   Off-hours Coverage _____

Phone Number _____

Email Address _____

Office Address _____

NOTES _____

_____

_____

_____

_____

_____

_____

_____

Doctor Name _____   Specialty _____

Assistant/PA Name _____   Off-hours Coverage _____

Phone Number _____

Email Address _____

Office Address _____

NOTES _____

_____

_____

_____

_____

_____

_____

Doctor Name _____   Specialty _____

Assistant/PA Name _____   Off-hours Coverage _____

Phone Number _____

Email Address _____

Office Address _____

NOTES _____

_____

_____

_____

_____

_____

Doctor Name .... Specialty ....

Assistant/PA Name .... Off-hours Coverage ....

Phone Number ....

Email Address ....

Office Address ....

NOTES ....

....

....

....

....

....

....

....

Doctor Name .... Specialty ....

Assistant/PA Name .... Off-hours Coverage ....

Phone Number ....

Email Address ....

Office Address ....

NOTES ....

....

....

....

....

....

....

PROBLEM SUMMARY LIST/ MEDICAL CONDITIONS

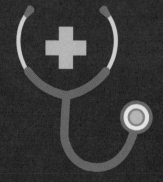

Copy and attach or list the summary of all medical conditions on these pages.

This list can be obtained from your physician or

from the patient portal from your provider.

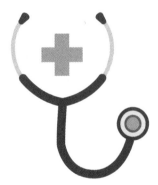

Copy and attach or list the summary of all medical conditions on these pages.

This list can be obtained from your physician or

from the patient portal from your provider.

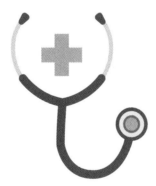

EVENT LOG

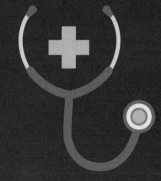

EVENT: ○ Appointment ○ ER/Urgent Care ○ Fall/Accident ○ Hospital

Date .... Doctor ....

Vitals .... Weight .... Blood Pressure ....

Reason for Visit ....

....

....

....

....

....

Notes ....

....

....

....

....

....

....

....

....

Follow-up ....

....

....

....

....

....

....

....

EVENT: ○ Appointment ○ ER/Urgent Care ○ Fall/Accident ○ Hospital

Date _____   Doctor _____

Vitals _____   Weight _____   Blood Pressure _____

Reason for Visit _____

_____

_____

_____

_____

_____

Notes _____

_____

_____

_____

_____

_____

_____

Follow-up _____

_____

_____

_____

_____

_____

EVENT: ○ Appointment ○ ER/Urgent Care ○ Fall/Accident ○ Hospital

Date _____   Doctor _____

Vitals _____   Weight _____   Blood Pressure _____

Reason for Visit _____

_____

_____

_____

_____

_____

_____

Notes _____

_____

_____

_____

_____

_____

_____

_____

_____

Follow-up _____

_____

_____

_____

_____

_____

_____

EVENT: ○ Appointment ○ ER/Urgent Care ○ Fall/Accident ○ Hospital

Date _____ Doctor _____

Vitals _____ Weight _____ Blood Pressure _____

Reason for Visit _____

_____

_____

_____

_____

Notes _____

_____

_____

_____

_____

_____

_____

Follow-up _____

_____

_____

_____

_____

_____

EVENT: o Appointment   o ER/Urgent Care   o Fall/Accident   o Hospital

Date _____   Doctor _____

Vitals _____   Weight _____   Blood Pressure _____

Reason for Visit _____

_____

_____

_____

_____

_____

Notes _____

_____

_____

_____

_____

_____

_____

_____

_____

Follow-up _____

_____

_____

_____

_____

_____

_____

_____

EVENT: ○ Appointment ○ ER/Urgent Care ○ Fall/Accident ○ Hospital

Date _____ Doctor _____

Vitals _____ Weight _____ Blood Pressure _____

Reason for Visit _____

_____

_____

_____

_____

_____

Notes _____

_____

_____

_____

_____

_____

_____

_____

Follow-up _____

_____

_____

_____

_____

_____

_____

EVENT: ○ Appointment   ○ ER/Urgent Care   ○ Fall/Accident   ○ Hospital

Date _____   Doctor _____

Vitals _____   Weight _____   Blood Pressure _____

Reason for Visit _____

_____

_____

_____

_____

_____

Notes _____

_____

_____

_____

_____

_____

_____

_____

Follow-up _____

_____

_____

_____

_____

_____

_____

EVENT: ○ Appointment ○ ER/Urgent Care ○ Fall/Accident ○ Hospital

Date _____   Doctor _____

Vitals _____   Weight _____   Blood Pressure _____

Reason for Visit _____

_____

_____

_____

_____

_____

_____

Notes _____

_____

_____

_____

_____

_____

_____

_____

_____

Follow-up _____

_____

_____

_____

_____

_____

_____

EVENT: ○ Appointment ○ ER/Urgent Care ○ Fall/Accident ○ Hospital

Date _____   Doctor _____

Vitals _____ Weight _____ Blood Pressure _____

Reason for Visit _____

_____

_____

_____

_____

Notes _____

_____

_____

_____

_____

_____

_____

Follow-up _____

_____

_____

_____

_____

_____

EVENT: ○ Appointment   ○ ER/Urgent Care   ○ Fall/Accident   ○ Hospital

Date _____   Doctor _____

Vitals _____   Weight _____   Blood Pressure _____

Reason for Visit _____

_____

_____

_____

_____

_____

Notes _____

_____

_____

_____

_____

_____

_____

_____

Follow-up _____

_____

_____

_____

_____

_____

EVENT: ○ Appointment ○ ER/Urgent Care ○ Fall/Accident ○ Hospital

Date _____ Doctor _____

Vitals _____ Weight _____ Blood Pressure _____

Reason for Visit _____

_____

_____

_____

_____

_____

Notes _____

_____

_____

_____

_____

_____

_____

_____

Follow-up _____

_____

_____

_____

_____

_____

_____

EVENT: ○ Appointment   ○ ER/Urgent Care   ○ Fall/Accident   ○ Hospital

Date _____   Doctor _____

Vitals _____   Weight _____   Blood Pressure _____

Reason for Visit _____

_____

_____

_____

_____

_____

Notes _____

_____

_____

_____

_____

_____

_____

_____

Follow-up _____

_____

_____

_____

_____

_____

_____

EVENT: ○ Appointment   ○ ER/Urgent Care   ○ Fall/Accident   ○ Hospital

Date ....   Doctor ....

Vitals ....   Weight ....   Blood Pressure ....

Reason for Visit ....

....

....

....

....

....

Notes ....

....

....

....

....

....

....

....

Follow-up ....

....

....

....

....

....

....

EVENT: ○ Appointment ○ ER/Urgent Care ○ Fall/Accident ○ Hospital

Date _____   Doctor _____

Vitals _____   Weight _____   Blood Pressure _____

Reason for Visit _____

_____

_____

_____

_____

Notes _____

_____

_____

_____

_____

_____

_____

Follow-up _____

_____

_____

_____

_____

_____

EVENT: ○ Appointment ○ ER/Urgent Care ○ Fall/Accident ○ Hospital

Date _____ Doctor _____

Vitals _____ Weight _____ Blood Pressure _____

Reason for Visit _____

_____

_____

_____

_____

_____

Notes _____

_____

_____

_____

_____

_____

_____

Follow-up _____

_____

_____

_____

_____

_____

_____

○ Appointment ○ ER/Urgent Care ○ Fall/Accident ○ Hospital

EVENT: ○ Appointment   ○ ER/Urgent Care   ○ Fall/Accident   ○ Hospital

Date _____   Doctor _____

Vitals _____   Weight _____   Blood Pressure _____

Reason for Visit _____

_____

_____

_____

_____

_____

Notes _____

_____

_____

_____

_____

_____

_____

_____

Follow-up _____

_____

_____

_____

_____

_____

_____

_____

EVENT: ○ Appointment   ○ ER/Urgent Care   ○ Fall/Accident   ○ Hospital

Date _____   Doctor _____

Vitals _____   Weight _____   Blood Pressure _____

Reason for Visit _____

_____

_____

_____

_____

_____

Notes _____

_____

_____

_____

_____

_____

_____

Follow-up _____

_____

_____

_____

_____

_____

_____

EVENT: ○ Appointment   ○ ER/Urgent Care   ○ Fall/Accident   ○ Hospital

Date _____   Doctor _____

Vitals _____   Weight _____   Blood Pressure _____

Reason for Visit _____

_____

_____

_____

_____

_____

Notes

_____

_____

_____

_____

_____

_____

_____

Follow-up _____

_____

_____

_____

_____

_____

_____

EVENT: ○ Appointment   ○ ER/Urgent Care   ○ Fall/Accident   ○ Hospital

Date _____   Doctor _____

Vitals _____   Weight _____   Blood Pressure _____

Reason for Visit _____

_____

_____

_____

_____

_____

_____

_____

Notes _____

_____

_____

_____

_____

_____

_____

_____

_____

_____

Follow-up _____

_____

_____

_____

_____

_____

_____

_____

○ Appointment   ○ ER/Urgent Care   ○ Fall/Accident   ○ Hospital

EVENT: ○ Appointment ○ ER/Urgent Care ○ Fall/Accident ○ Hospital

Date _____ Doctor _____

Vitals _____ Weight _____ Blood Pressure _____

Reason for Visit _____

_____

_____

_____

_____

_____

Notes _____

_____

_____

_____

_____

_____

_____

Follow-up _____

_____

_____

_____

_____

_____

EVENT: ○ Appointment   ○ ER/Urgent Care   ○ Fall/Accident   ○ Hospital

Date _____   Doctor _____

Vitals _____   Weight _____   Blood Pressure _____

Reason for Visit _____

_____

_____

_____

_____

_____

Notes _____

_____

_____

_____

_____

_____

Follow-up _____

_____

_____

_____

_____

_____

○ Appointment   ○ ER/Urgent Care   ○ Fall/Accident   ○ Hospital

EVENT:　○ Appointment　○ ER/Urgent Care　○ Fall/Accident　○ Hospital

Date _____　Doctor _____

Vitals _____　Weight _____　Blood Pressure _____

Reason for Visit _____

_____

_____

_____

_____

_____

Notes _____

_____

_____

_____

_____

_____

_____

_____

Follow-up _____

_____

_____

_____

_____

_____

_____

EVENT: ○ Appointment ○ ER/Urgent Care ○ Fall/Accident ○ Hospital

Date _____   Doctor _____

Vitals _____   Weight _____   Blood Pressure _____

Reason for Visit _____

_____

_____

_____

_____

Notes _____

_____

_____

_____

_____

_____

_____

_____

Follow-up _____

_____

_____

_____

_____

_____

_____

EVENT:

○ Appointment   ○ ER/Urgent Care   ○ Fall/Accident   ○ Hospital

Date _____   Doctor _____

Vitals _____   Weight _____   Blood Pressure _____

Reason for Visit _____

_____

_____

_____

_____

_____

Notes _____

_____

_____

_____

_____

_____

_____

_____

_____

Follow-up _____

_____

_____

_____

_____

_____

_____

_____

_____

EVENT: ○ Appointment ○ ER/Urgent Care ○ Fall/Accident ○ Hospital

Date _____   Doctor _____

Vitals _____   Weight _____   Blood Pressure _____

Reason for Visit _____

_____

_____

_____

_____

_____

_____

Notes _____

_____

_____

_____

_____

_____

_____

_____

Follow-up _____

_____

_____

_____

_____

_____

_____

EVENT: ○ Appointment   ○ ER/Urgent Care   ○ Fall/Accident   ○ Hospital

Date _____   Doctor _____

Vitals _____   Weight _____   Blood Pressure _____

Reason for Visit _____

_____

_____

_____

_____

Notes _____

_____

_____

_____

_____

_____

_____

_____

Follow-up _____

_____

_____

_____

_____

_____

_____

EVENT: ○ Appointment   ○ ER/Urgent Care   ○ Fall/Accident   ○ Hospital

Date _____   Doctor _____

Vitals _____   Weight _____   Blood Pressure _____

Reason for Visit _____

_____

_____

_____

_____

_____

Notes _____

_____

_____

_____

_____

_____

_____

_____

Follow-up _____

_____

_____

_____

_____

_____

_____

_____

EVENT: ○ Appointment ○ ER/Urgent Care ○ Fall/Accident ○ Hospital

Date .... Doctor ....

Vitals .... Weight .... Blood Pressure ....

Reason for Visit ....

....

....

....

....

....

Notes ....

....

....

....

....

....

....

....

Follow-up ....

....

....

....

....

....

....

....

EVENT: ○ Appointment   ○ ER/Urgent Care   ○ Fall/Accident   ○ Hospital

Date _____   Doctor _____

Vitals _____   Weight _____   Blood Pressure _____

Reason for Visit _____

_____

_____

_____

_____

Notes _____

_____

_____

_____

_____

_____

_____

_____

Follow-up _____

_____

_____

_____

_____

_____

_____

EVENT: ○ Appointment ○ ER/Urgent Care ○ Fall/Accident ○ Hospital

Date _____ Doctor _____

Vitals _____ Weight _____ Blood Pressure _____

Reason for Visit _____

_____

_____

_____

_____

Notes _____

_____

_____

_____

_____

_____

_____

Follow-up _____

_____

_____

_____

_____

_____

EVENT:　○ Appointment　○ ER/Urgent Care　○ Fall/Accident　○ Hospital

Date _____　Doctor _____

Vitals _____　Weight _____　Blood Pressure _____

Reason for Visit _____

_____

_____

_____

_____

_____

Notes _____

_____

_____

_____

_____

_____

_____

_____

Follow-up _____

_____

_____

_____

_____

_____

_____

EVENT: ○ Appointment   ○ ER/Urgent Care   ○ Fall/Accident   ○ Hospital

Date _____   Doctor _____

Vitals _____   Weight _____   Blood Pressure _____

Reason for Visit _____

_____

_____

_____

_____

_____

Notes _____

_____

_____

_____

_____

_____

_____

_____

_____

Follow-up _____

_____

_____

_____

_____

_____

_____

EVENT: ○ Appointment ○ ER/Urgent Care ○ Fall/Accident ○ Hospital

Date _____ Doctor _____

Vitals _____ Weight _____ Blood Pressure _____

Reason for Visit _____

_____

_____

_____

_____

Notes _____

_____

_____

_____

_____

_____

_____

Follow-up _____

_____

_____

_____

_____

_____

EVENT: ○ Appointment ○ ER/Urgent Care ○ Fall/Accident ○ Hospital

Date _____ Doctor _____

Vitals _____ Weight _____ Blood Pressure _____

Reason for Visit _____

_____

_____

_____

_____

_____

Notes _____

_____

_____

_____

_____

_____

_____

_____

_____

Follow-up _____

_____

_____

_____

_____

_____

_____

EVENT: ○ Appointment   ○ ER/Urgent Care   ○ Fall/Accident   ○ Hospital

Date _____   Doctor _____

Vitals _____   Weight _____   Blood Pressure _____

Reason for Visit _____

_____

_____

_____

_____

_____

Notes _____

_____

_____

_____

_____

_____

_____

_____

Follow-up _____

_____

_____

_____

_____

_____

_____

EVENT: ○ Appointment   ○ ER/Urgent Care   ○ Fall/Accident   ○ Hospital

Date _____   Doctor _____

Vitals _____   Weight _____   Blood Pressure _____

Reason for Visit _____

_____

_____

_____

_____

_____

_____

Notes _____

_____

_____

_____

_____

_____

_____

_____

_____

Follow-up _____

_____

_____

_____

_____

_____

_____

_____

EVENT: ○ Appointment   ○ ER/Urgent Care   ○ Fall/Accident   ○ Hospital

Date _____   Doctor _____

Vitals _____   Weight _____   Blood Pressure _____

Reason for Visit _____

_____

_____

_____

_____

_____

_____

Notes _____

_____

_____

_____

_____

_____

_____

_____

_____

_____

Follow-up _____

_____

_____

_____

_____

_____

_____

_____

EVENT: ○ Appointment ○ ER/Urgent Care ○ Fall/Accident ○ Hospital

Date _____   Doctor _____

Vitals _____   Weight _____   Blood Pressure _____

Reason for Visit _____

_____

_____

_____

_____

Notes _____

_____

_____

_____

_____

_____

_____

_____

Follow-up _____

_____

_____

_____

_____

_____

_____

EVENT: ○ Appointment ○ ER/Urgent Care ○ Fall/Accident ○ Hospital

Date _____   Doctor _____

Vitals _____   Weight _____   Blood Pressure _____

Reason for Visit _____

_____

_____

_____

_____

_____

Notes _____

_____

_____

_____

_____

_____

_____

Follow-up _____

_____

_____

_____

_____

_____

EVENT: ○ Appointment ○ ER/Urgent Care ○ Fall/Accident ○ Hospital

Date _____ Doctor _____

Vitals _____ Weight _____ Blood Pressure _____

Reason for Visit _____

_____

_____

_____

_____

_____

Notes _____

_____

_____

_____

_____

_____

_____

_____

Follow-up _____

_____

_____

_____

_____

_____

_____

MEDICATION RECORD

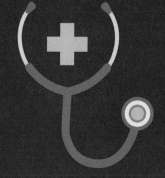

Medication Name & Dose _____

o With food   o Without food   **AM   MidDay   PM   Bedtime**

Prescribed by _____

Date Prescribed _____   Date Ended _____

Prescribed for _____

Side Effects _____

_____

Time to take effect (see results) _____

Medication Name & Dose _____

o With food   o Without food   **AM   MidDay   PM   Bedtime**

Prescribed by _____

Date Prescribed _____   Date Ended _____

Prescribed for _____

Side Effects _____

_____

Time to take effect (see results) _____

Medication Name & Dose _____

o With food   o Without food   **AM   MidDay   PM   Bedtime**

Prescribed by _____

Date Prescribed _____   Date Ended _____

Prescribed for _____

Side Effects _____

_____

Time to take effect (see results) _____

Medication Name & Dose _____

○ With food   ○ Without food   **AM   MidDay   PM   Bedtime**

Prescribed by _____

Date Prescribed _____ Date Ended _____

Prescribed for _____

Side Effects _____

_____

Time to take effect (see results) _____

Medication Name & Dose _____

○ With food   ○ Without food   **AM   MidDay   PM   Bedtime**

Prescribed by _____

Date Prescribed _____ Date Ended _____

Prescribed for _____

Side Effects _____

_____

Time to take effect (see results) _____

Medication Name & Dose _____

○ With food   ○ Without food   **AM   MidDay   PM   Bedtime**

Prescribed by _____

Date Prescribed _____ Date Ended _____

Prescribed for _____

Side Effects _____

_____

Time to take effect (see results) _____

Medication Name & Dose _____

○ With food   ○ Without food   **AM   MidDay   PM   Bedtime**

Prescribed by _____

Date Prescribed _____ Date Ended _____

Prescribed for _____

Side Effects _____

_____

Time to take effect (see results) _____

Medication Name & Dose _____

○ With food   ○ Without food   **AM   MidDay   PM   Bedtime**

Prescribed by _____

Date Prescribed _____ Date Ended _____

Prescribed for _____

Side Effects _____

_____

Time to take effect (see results) _____

Medication Name & Dose _____

○ With food   ○ Without food   **AM   MidDay   PM   Bedtime**

Prescribed by _____

Date Prescribed _____ Date Ended _____

Prescribed for _____

Side Effects _____

_____

Time to take effect (see results) _____

Medication Name & Dose _____

○ With food   ○ Without food   **AM   MidDay   PM   Bedtime**

Prescribed by _____

Date Prescribed _____   Date Ended _____

Prescribed for _____

Side Effects _____

_____

Time to take effect (see results) _____

Medication Name & Dose _____

○ With food   ○ Without food   **AM   MidDay   PM   Bedtime**

Prescribed by _____

Date Prescribed _____   Date Ended _____

Prescribed for _____

Side Effects _____

_____

Time to take effect (see results) _____

Medication Name & Dose _____

○ With food   ○ Without food   **AM   MidDay   PM   Bedtime**

Prescribed by _____

Date Prescribed _____   Date Ended _____

Prescribed for _____

Side Effects _____

_____

Time to take effect (see results) _____

Medication Name & Dose _____

○ With food   ○ Without food   **AM   MidDay   PM   Bedtime**

Prescribed by _____

Date Prescribed _____ Date Ended _____

Prescribed for _____

Side Effects _____

_____

Time to take effect (see results) _____

Medication Name & Dose _____

○ With food   ○ Without food   **AM   MidDay   PM   Bedtime**

Prescribed by _____

Date Prescribed _____ Date Ended _____

Prescribed for _____

Side Effects _____

_____

Time to take effect (see results) _____

Medication Name & Dose _____

○ With food   ○ Without food   **AM   MidDay   PM   Bedtime**

Prescribed by _____

Date Prescribed _____ Date Ended _____

Prescribed for _____

Side Effects _____

_____

Time to take effect (see results) _____

Medication Name & Dose _____

○ With food   ○ Without food   **AM**   **MidDay**   **PM**   **Bedtime**

Prescribed by _____

Date Prescribed _____   Date Ended _____

Prescribed for _____

Side Effects _____

_____

Time to take effect (see results) _____

Medication Name & Dose _____

○ With food   ○ Without food   **AM**   **MidDay**   **PM**   **Bedtime**

Prescribed by _____

Date Prescribed _____   Date Ended _____

Prescribed for _____

Side Effects _____

_____

Time to take effect (see results) _____

Medication Name & Dose _____

○ With food   ○ Without food   **AM**   **MidDay**   **PM**   **Bedtime**

Prescribed by _____

Date Prescribed _____   Date Ended _____

Prescribed for _____

Side Effects _____

_____

Time to take effect (see results) _____

Medication Name & Dose _____

○ With food   ○ Without food   **AM   MidDay   PM   Bedtime**

Prescribed by _____

Date Prescribed _____ Date Ended _____

Prescribed for _____

Side Effects _____

_____

Time to take effect (see results) _____

Medication Name & Dose _____

○ With food   ○ Without food   **AM   MidDay   PM   Bedtime**

Prescribed by _____

Date Prescribed _____ Date Ended _____

Prescribed for _____

Side Effects _____

_____

Time to take effect (see results) _____

Medication Name & Dose _____

○ With food   ○ Without food   **AM   MidDay   PM   Bedtime**

Prescribed by _____

Date Prescribed _____ Date Ended _____

Prescribed for _____

Side Effects _____

_____

Time to take effect (see results) _____

Medication Name & Dose _____

○ With food   ○ Without food   **AM**   **MidDay**   **PM**   **Bedtime**

Prescribed by _____

Date Prescribed _____   Date Ended _____

Prescribed for _____

Side Effects _____

_____

Time to take effect (see results) _____

Medication Name & Dose _____

○ With food   ○ Without food   **AM**   **MidDay**   **PM**   **Bedtime**

Prescribed by _____

Date Prescribed _____   Date Ended _____

Prescribed for _____

Side Effects _____

_____

Time to take effect (see results) _____

Medication Name & Dose _____

○ With food   ○ Without food   **AM**   **MidDay**   **PM**   **Bedtime**

Prescribed by _____

Date Prescribed _____   Date Ended _____

Prescribed for _____

Side Effects _____

_____

Time to take effect (see results) _____

SUPPLEMENTS, HERBALS, VITAMINS, ETC.

Name	Dose	Date Started	Date Ended

SUPPLEMENTS, HERBALS, VITAMINS, ETC.

Name	Dose	Date Started	Date Ended

ALLERGY RECORD

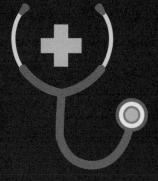

Allergic to _____

Generic Name _____

Prescribed for _____

Reaction _____

Allergic to _____

Generic Name _____

Prescribed for _____

Reaction _____

Allergic to _____

Generic Name _____

Prescribed for _____

Reaction _____

Allergic to _____

Generic Name _____

Prescribed for _____

Reaction _____

Allergic to _____

Generic Name _____

Prescribed for _____

Reaction _____

Allergic to _____

Generic Name _____

Prescribed for _____

Reaction _____

Allergic to _____

Generic Name _____

Prescribed for _____

Reaction _____

Allergic to _____

Generic Name _____

Prescribed for _____

Reaction _____

Allergic to _____

Generic Name _____

Prescribed for _____

Reaction _____

Allergic to _____

Generic Name _____

Prescribed for _____

Reaction _____

THERAPY
RECORD

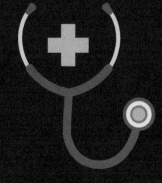

Therapy Type ....

Prescribed by ....

Provider .... Frequency ....

Date Prescribed .... Date Ended ....

Prescribed for ....

Side Effects to watch for ....

....

Time to take effect (see results) ....

Therapy Type ....

Prescribed by ....

Provider .... Frequency ....

Date Prescribed .... Date Ended ....

Prescribed for ....

Side Effects to watch for ....

....

Time to take effect (see results) ....

Therapy Type ....

Prescribed by ....

Provider .... Frequency ....

Date Prescribed .... Date Ended ....

Prescribed for ....

Side Effects to watch for ....

....

Time to take effect (see results) ....

Therapy Type _____

Prescribed by _____

Provider _____ Frequency _____

Date Prescribed _____ Date Ended _____

Prescribed for _____

Side Effects to watch for _____

_____

Time to take effect (see results) _____

Therapy Type _____

Prescribed by _____

Provider _____ Frequency _____

Date Prescribed _____ Date Ended _____

Prescribed for _____

Side Effects to watch for _____

_____

Time to take effect (see results) _____

Therapy Type _____

Prescribed by _____

Provider _____ Frequency _____

Date Prescribed _____ Date Ended _____

Prescribed for _____

Side Effects to watch for _____

_____

Time to take effect (see results) _____

Therapy Type

Prescribed by

Provider _____ Frequency

Date Prescribed _____ Date Ended

Prescribed for

Side Effects to watch for

Time to take effect (see results)

Therapy Type

Prescribed by

Provider _____ Frequency

Date Prescribed _____ Date Ended

Prescribed for

Side Effects to watch for

Time to take effect (see results)

Therapy Type

Prescribed by

Provider _____ Frequency

Date Prescribed _____ Date Ended

Prescribed for

Side Effects to watch for

Time to take effect (see results)

Therapy Type ....

Prescribed by ....

Provider .... Frequency ....

Date Prescribed .... Date Ended ....

Prescribed for ....

Side Effects to watch for ....

....

Time to take effect (see results) ....

Therapy Type ....

Prescribed by ....

Provider .... Frequency ....

Date Prescribed .... Date Ended ....

Prescribed for ....

Side Effects to watch for ....

....

Time to take effect (see results) ....

Therapy Type ....

Prescribed by ....

Provider .... Frequency ....

Date Prescribed .... Date Ended ....

Prescribed for ....

Side Effects to watch for ....

....

Time to take effect (see results) ....

Therapy Type _____

Prescribed by _____

Provider _____ Frequency _____

Date Prescribed _____ Date Ended _____

Prescribed for _____

Side Effects to watch for _____

_____

Time to take effect (see results) _____

Therapy Type _____

Prescribed by _____

Provider _____ Frequency _____

Date Prescribed _____ Date Ended _____

Prescribed for _____

Side Effects to watch for _____

_____

Time to take effect (see results) _____

Therapy Type _____

Prescribed by _____

Provider _____ Frequency _____

Date Prescribed _____ Date Ended _____

Prescribed for _____

Side Effects to watch for _____

_____

Time to take effect (see results) _____

Therapy Type _____

Prescribed by _____

Provider _____ Frequency _____

Date Prescribed _____ Date Ended _____

Prescribed for _____

Side Effects to watch for _____

_____

Time to take effect (see results) _____

Therapy Type _____

Prescribed by _____

Provider _____ Frequency _____

Date Prescribed _____ Date Ended _____

Prescribed for _____

Side Effects to watch for _____

_____

Time to take effect (see results) _____

Therapy Type _____

Prescribed by _____

Provider _____ Frequency _____

Date Prescribed _____ Date Ended _____

Prescribed for _____

Side Effects to watch for _____

_____

Time to take effect (see results) _____

Therapy Type _____

Prescribed by _____

Provider _____ Frequency _____

Date Prescribed _____ Date Ended _____

Prescribed for _____

Side Effects to watch for _____

_____

Time to take effect (see results) _____

Therapy Type _____

Prescribed by _____

Provider _____ Frequency _____

Date Prescribed _____ Date Ended _____

Prescribed for _____

Side Effects to watch for _____

_____

Time to take effect (see results) _____

Therapy Type _____

Prescribed by _____

Provider _____ Frequency _____

Date Prescribed _____ Date Ended _____

Prescribed for _____

Side Effects to watch for _____

_____

Time to take effect (see results) _____

Therapy Type ....

Prescribed by ....

Provider .... Frequency ....

Date Prescribed .... Date Ended ....

Prescribed for ....

Side Effects to watch for ....

....

Time to take effect (see results) ....

Therapy Type ....

Prescribed by ....

Provider .... Frequency ....

Date Prescribed .... Date Ended ....

Prescribed for ....

Side Effects to watch for ....

....

Time to take effect (see results) ....

Therapy Type ....

Prescribed by ....

Provider .... Frequency ....

Date Prescribed .... Date Ended ....

Prescribed for ....

Side Effects to watch for ....

....

Time to take effect (see results) ....

Therapy Type _____

Prescribed by _____

Provider _____ Frequency _____

Date Prescribed _____ Date Ended _____

Prescribed for _____

Side Effects to watch for _____

_____

Time to take effect (see results) _____

Therapy Type _____

Prescribed by _____

Provider _____ Frequency _____

Date Prescribed _____ Date Ended _____

Prescribed for _____

Side Effects to watch for _____

_____

Time to take effect (see results) _____

Therapy Type _____

Prescribed by _____

Provider _____ Frequency _____

Date Prescribed _____ Date Ended _____

Prescribed for _____

Side Effects to watch for _____

_____

Time to take effect (see results) _____

Therapy Type ....

Prescribed by ....

Provider .... Frequency ....

Date Prescribed .... Date Ended ....

Prescribed for ....

Side Effects to watch for ....

....

Time to take effect (see results) ....

Therapy Type ....

Prescribed by ....

Provider .... Frequency ....

Date Prescribed .... Date Ended ....

Prescribed for ....

Side Effects to watch for ....

....

Time to take effect (see results) ....

Therapy Type ....

Prescribed by ....

Provider .... Frequency ....

Date Prescribed .... Date Ended ....

Prescribed for ....

Side Effects to watch for ....

....

Time to take effect (see results) ....

SURGERY
RECORD

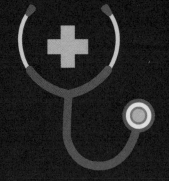

Date

Surgery/Procedure

Doctor

Results/Notes

Date

Surgery/Procedure

Doctor

Results/Notes

Date

Surgery/Procedure

Doctor

Results/Notes

Date

Surgery/Procedure

Doctor

Results/Notes

Date

Surgery/Procedure

Doctor

Results/Notes

Date ....

Surgery/Procedure ....

Doctor ....

Results/Notes ....

Date ....

Surgery/Procedure ....

Doctor ....

Results/Notes ....

Date ....

Surgery/Procedure ....

Doctor ....

Results/Notes ....

Date ....

Surgery/Procedure ....

Doctor ....

Results/Notes ....

Date ....

Surgery/Procedure ....

Doctor ....

Results/Notes ....

Date _____

Surgery/Procedure _____

Doctor _____

Results/Notes _____

Date _____

Surgery/Procedure _____

Doctor _____

Results/Notes _____

Date _____

Surgery/Procedure _____

Doctor _____

Results/Notes _____

Date _____

Surgery/Procedure _____

Doctor _____

Results/Notes _____

Date _____

Surgery/Procedure _____

Doctor _____

Results/Notes _____

Date

Surgery/Procedure

Doctor

Results/Notes

Date

Surgery/Procedure

Doctor

Results/Notes

Date

Surgery/Procedure

Doctor

Results/Notes

Date

Surgery/Procedure

Doctor

Results/Notes

Date

Surgery/Procedure

Doctor

Results/Notes

Date

Surgery/Procedure

Doctor

Results/Notes

Date

Surgery/Procedure

Doctor

Results/Notes

Date

Surgery/Procedure

Doctor

Results/Notes

Date

Surgery/Procedure

Doctor

Results/Notes

Date

Surgery/Procedure

Doctor

Results/Notes

Date _____

Surgery/Procedure _____

Doctor _____

Results/Notes _____

Date _____

Surgery/Procedure _____

Doctor _____

Results/Notes _____

Date _____

Surgery/Procedure _____

Doctor _____

Results/Notes _____

Date _____

Surgery/Procedure _____

Doctor _____

Results/Notes _____

Date _____

Surgery/Procedure _____

Doctor _____

Results/Notes _____

NEGOTIATING MEDICAL BILLS

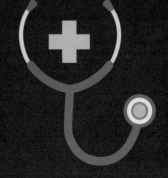

How to Negotiate Medical Bills

Always keep meticulous records of each contact. For every call: the name of the representative you spoke with, the date of the conversation, what agreement was made, always get a direct call back number for that person.

Getting a doctor, hospital, or other medical provider to discount or write down a bill, or to offer a payment plan, may not be as difficult as you think. Under the Affordable Care Act, nonprofit hospitals are required to have a Financial Assistance Policy (FAP) for patients who are unable to afford their care—or the hospital risks losing their tax-exempt status. This policy includes free or discounted care. The exemptions for FAPs are dictated by the IRS Section 501(r)(4).

Assistance varies by geographic area and by provider. Assistance can take the form of writing-off a bill, writing-down a bill, lump-sum payment, discount charity care, or payment plans. You can search "Name of hospital + financial assistance" to find out the policies and criteria for your specific facility.

Follow these steps to help improve the odds for a positive outcome.

BEFORE medical services have been provided - steps to take

1. Contact the billing office of the provider.

2. Explain your financial situation (be honest and realistic about what you can afford to pay).

3. Ask about all assistance options available.

   - *Write-offs (the provider reduces the bill to $0)*

   - *Write-downs (the provider writes off a large portion of the bill)*

   - *Lump sum discounts for paying the entire bill (20% is common, but you can ask for more)*

   - Consider payment plans (be realistic about what you can afford monthly and set that amount before negotiating).

Under the Affordable Care Act, non-profit hospitals
are required to offer patient assistance programs

AFTER medical services have been provided - steps to take

1. Request an itemized bill.

2. Make sure all the bills are accounted for before beginning the negotiation process.

3. When speaking with the billing department, ask that your bill be "**put on hold from collections**" and that your account status be updated to "**pending**".

4. Ask about any hardship program or charity care that is available.

5. Apply first before paying—do it soon. Sometimes there is a ninety-day limit.

Under the Affordable Care Act, non-profit hospitals
are required to offer patient assistance programs

The Negotiation Process

1. Review the itemized bill.

   - *If you're discharged in the morning (as most patients are), dispute if you're charged with a full daily-room rate for the date you left the hospital.*

   - *Dispute any additional fees on the bill for routine supplies, like gowns, gloves or sheets. These items should be factored into the hospital daily-room charge, because they are "considered the cost of doing business."*

2. If you are able to pay the bill on one lump-sum, request a discount.

- *Your doctor, hospital, clinic, or therapy provider may offer a pay-in-full discount.*

- *A discount is more likely with a collection service or vendor who has purchased the debt. NOTE: Having a bill sent to collections will impact your credit score. It is always best to avoid this happening.*

- *A 20% discount is common.*

3. Show evidence of cheaper service.

   - *Refer to the* Healthcare Bluebook *to compare your charges with national averages.*

   - *Check the Medicare price at* www.cms.gov.

   - clearhealthcosts.com/useful-links/#US-Government-price-lists

   - fairhealthconsumer.org/

   - Ask about a payment plan.

     - *Calculate how much you can realistically afford to pay monthly before beginning negotiations.*

     - *Request no interest or very low interest be charged.*

     - *Get details of the payment plan in writing.*

     - *Once a plan has been agreed upon, keep current on your payments. If you fall behind, the agreement may be voided.*

     - *If your situation changes and you are not able to make a payment, contact the billing office immediately to discuss options.*

For many years Sourcebooks has proudly supported Binc and continue this commitment with the publishing of this journal. Binc's mission is to strengthen the bookselling and comic retail community through charitable programs that support employees and their families. Their core program provides assistance to employees and shop owners who have a demonstrated financial need arising from severe hardship and/or emergency circumstances. Since the Foundation's inception in 1996, the organization has provided thousands of families with financial assistance, scholarships, and other emergency resources. Support for the Foundation's programs and services comes from all sectors of the book and comic industries. The Foundation was imagined and built by booksellers and proudly continues to be their safety net.

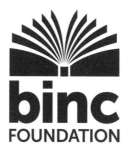

To find out more about the Binc Foundation,

please visit http://bincfoundation.org